PANDEMIC 2020
A 9 Year Old's Perspective

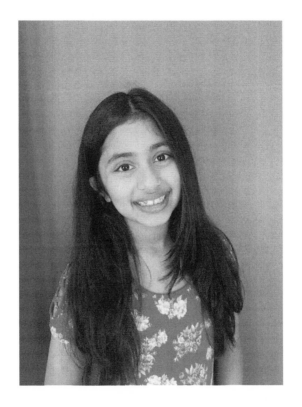

Practical Tips for Online School, Hobbies, and Healthy Habits during Covid-19

PRISHA HEDAU

PANDEMIC 2020
A 9 Year Old's Perspective

©2020 Prisha Hedau

print ISBN: 978-1-09832-875-7
ebook ISBN: 978-1-09832-876-4

Book design and printed by Bookbaby
Global Distribution by Bookbaby

CONTENTS

INTRODUCTION   1

THANK YOU   3

CHAPTER 1:MY LIFE BEFORE COVID-19   5

CHAPTER 2: THE BEGINNING OF A PANDEMIC   8

CHAPTER 3: CHANGING PERSPECTIVE   11

CHAPTER 4: IMPACTS DURING LOCKDOWN   14

CHAPTER 5: THINGS TO DO DURING QUARANTINE   23

CHAPTER 6: TIPS FOR ONLINE SCHOOLING   30

CHAPTER 7: FOCUS ON THE POSITIVE THINGS   33

CHAPTER 8: LESSONS LEARNT   37

CHAPTER 9: LOOKING AHEAD   40

CHAPTER 10: BE GRATEFUL   42

INTRODUCTION

Hi readers! I'm Prisha, from Louisville, Kentucky. I am your author for this book. These are challenging times. This is a different book, and a different story—that's why it's unique. I'm sure that a whole new perspective will be shown.

I am writing this book to share my feelings, thoughts, and learnings from this pandemic. It all started by writing daily notes to remember my experience during a pandemic. One evening, my parents suggested I start writing a book instead of just note cards. Soon I became interested in writing a book of my own. I wanted to write this book to share with others the useful tips for online school, hobbies, and healthy habits. I also wanted to write a book as a memory that can be referred to in the future. I believe a book is the most valuable object for reference and something special that one can ever receive. I'd also like to share what I think and my perspective with you.

Okay, enough talk about this book or I will tell you everything at once.

Here is a little bit about me, I'm starting fifth grade this August, 2020-2021. I am an author, singer, swimmer, dancer, painter, player, friend, a family member, etc. By the way, if you are wondering—yes, I am nine years old, but will turn ten by the end of September. So first off, I do dance, which is something that makes me happy and is something that I'm good at. If I forgot to mention, I proudly own my own YouTube channel, named Prisha Hedau. It's titled after my name. I know, it is a little boring, but it makes a statement.

Hmm, let's see,. I also love math and science, presenting, and confidently speaking. Well, that's more than enough. Feel free to turn the page. Hope you'll enjoy this book!

THANK YOU

I would like to thank my parents (Rajendra Hedau and Rachana Pandey) for being who they are, and supporting in every way possible. They have shown me how much they care about me and our family throughout this crazy time that has still not ended. Adding to that, I would also like to thank all of my teachers who gave me support and knowledge to this day and especially my fourth-grade teachers for doing a lot for us, especially at the end of the year when the pandemic started.

During this Pandemic, some very important people were there for us and the whole world. Can you guess who they are? Essential workers and First Responders! You got that right. If they didn't do what they were doing, and still to this day don't do what they are doing, we would be so far lost and hurt. We appreciate you! In addition to that, we appreciate everybody who is doing their part to keep them, their loved ones, and their community safe. Thank you everyone!

CHAPTER 1:
MY LIFE BEFORE COVID-19

See, life before a pandemic was better than life in a pandemic, though I probably wouldn't know that was correct back at the time in my normal life. I didn't even know what the word "Pandemic" meant. I am not joking! Now, the word "pandemic" is the word of the year. What have you done, 2020? I thought my life was absolutely boring. Well...I was wrong. FYI, it is also somewhat nice to have experienced a pandemic in life, because it has taught me so much and opened a whole new perspective to me.

I am thankful—not fully, but I still am somewhat thankful—for having this once-in-a-lifetime experience to appreciate what I have in my life and for what I am most grateful.

Here's a sample of my life before a pandemic. Good morning Prisha, it's time for another ordinary day. As

I woke up, I would be half awake and half asleep and I would do my daily morning to-do things including: brushing my teeth, doing my hair, skin care, and taking a bath. After that, I would get nicely dressed and go downstairs for breakfast. Often times, I watched something on the computer while I ate. By the time I finished breakfast, my parents would be packing up to leave the house. We all would be out of the house by 8:15 am. We sat in the car and went through everyday traffic, which I can proudly say was something I disliked the most in a normal day, in my normal life. After crazy traffic, I would go to school. By 3:45 pm, I would be in CEP (an after-school program) until my parents picked me up. If you don't know what CEP is, well it's somewhere you stay until your parents come to pick you up. You can play, do homework, or talk with a friend. I go to CEP because my parents work all the way in downtown Louisville, and have to work until 5:00 pm. It takes them one-hour to drive to come pick me up. I don't have a problem with that, because I understand. This is off-topic! When they arrived to pick me up, we would either go straight home after CEP, or we would go to any of my after-school activities (for example, math classes, swimming, dancing, and other ones that I enjoy). After a long day, we all would come home, eat dinner, watch some TV, go to bed, and do the same all over again the next day.

On the weekends, it would be more fun activities, such as going to the mall, sleepovers, movie night, eating out, and friends and family gatherings. That's basically how my whole week went, from getting up at 7:30 am, to having sleepovers and talking almost all night.

CHAPTER 2:
THE BEGINNING OF A PANDEMIC

In the beginning of March, I was at school. Around 3:45 pm, when the school bell rang as I was walking to CEP (after school child enrichment program), I suddenly noticed my mom standing there. I had a mix of feelings— confusion, excitement, and one that I can't explain, and I bet you are wondering why. Well, so was I. My mom came two hours early from her work, just for me? For what reason? That was something I didn't know. So, I asked her. What else was I supposed to do? We walked to the car as she explained her choice of action. Here is the summary of what she said. "From that day until some point in the future, I won't go to work and you will not be going to school. We will work from home (WFH) because there is a COVID-19 POSITIVE CASE in Louisville."

"Oh, okay." I said. I was excited and scared and confused. I was excited because I finally get time to relax in the day. Let me tell you that on my normal day in my life, I would have nonstop things to do and the only time I could relax was late in the evening around 8:00 pm and only for maybe thirty to sixty minutes. Dinner time was late at night around 7:45 pm, and I am not complaining. I am just saying that I barely had any time to relax and ended up embracing the whole experience all over again the next day. So yes, I was happy to have all day to myself. I was also quite scared and confused. I have cousins who live around the world, including Europe. In their area in Europe, in the beginning of the pandemic it was really bad and scary for them as somehow virus was spreading fast in their country. When we would call them, it would seem scary, sad, and boring. It was different than previous calls full of fun. If that was the feeling there, wouldn't it be similar to the feeling we would get in Louisville? It's scary that it's spreading in Louisville (where I live) already, but on the bright side, I get to stay at home. I thought this meant life was going to be easy. Oh boy, was I wrong. I was just about to figure that out in ninety-six hours (four days!) This stuff was serious— it was the beginning of a whole pandemic! I had many questions. What was going to happen next? When will it end? How long will the pandemic last? I am no magic creature who can see the future, so I somehow just went along with the flow, not knowing what was going to happen next. All of these questions came to me when I watched—and sometimes still watch— Kentucky's news in the television. The Spanish Flu (flu) and COVID-19 (coronavirus) are two different viruses that affected people in two different ways, though they are spread in the same way. If you're wondering on how it spreads, this is a basic explanation. In one area, a person gets infected and a certain someone (it could be anyone) goes to that area and brings it back to his hometown. Then, then it spreads in that town and someone else comes to that area.............and so on, so forth. See, I know a little about life - I would like to share my thoughts with you as we go forward in this book.

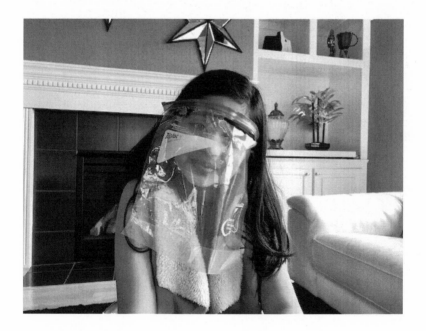

CHAPTER 3:
CHANGING PERSPECTIVE

There is a path you're given, and you have to be smart to pick the right one. In life, love, disappointment, trust, excitement, success, and failure comes and other things may come too. What I'm talking about here has another meaning to it—if you've been successful, then you have been through failure, and if you've been excited, then you have been through disappointment. Likewise, Covid-19 brought unexpected times where we can't do much. Sometimes, when life spares consequences, you must accept them and move on, or else it will consume you. Adding to that, there are times in life were you've just got to embrace what you can because everything won't always go as planned. This is one of those time – Accept and Embrace! You know, I can go on and on if you hand me a topic. If you want proof, ask my mom (I already gave you some proof). I bet she would say that I always have a lot to offer (most of the time that's right). If you're wondering why I know this much, I'm not really the person to ask because honestly, I have no clue. I am just a simple, unique, and chill fourth grader with apparently a ton to offer and I will give it to you because you're not wrong.

By the way, as we are speaking about perspectives, my perspective towards life is to have fun and be happy. What are your favorite events in life? I obviously won't be able to figure out yours, but you can figure out mine. One of my favorite events in our life is probably New Years' Eves. We have created a family tradition to spend New Year's Eve night with friends, blaring music, games, and excitement. I love the countdown. It is just so nice and fun, like, a whole new year and a whole new beginning, starting off with—drum roll please—cake, sleepovers, and my favorite part, no clocks or watches to remind us what time it is and I am being real here. A few of the families who come over would stay to talk and chill and we would "talk and chill" until one am!!!! It was a lot of fun. My birthday is something I also enjoy very much. If you noticed, I just like simple and fun gatherings with simple and fun people. By fun, I mean the crazy and hyper type. Let me tell you, the family of my own who lives in Kentucky is not so simple. As much as we act simple, we are...well, I can't really explain, but I can give you an example. My mom, she gets a little emotional when she watch movies. To the people out there who are not emotional—dude, I am so with you. I never understand the need to cry in a movie that is funny, romantic, sad, or a hit. My mom loves watching movies in Hindi, and it also has to be during her college time movie of hers?

WARNING/this book will be filled with Emotions

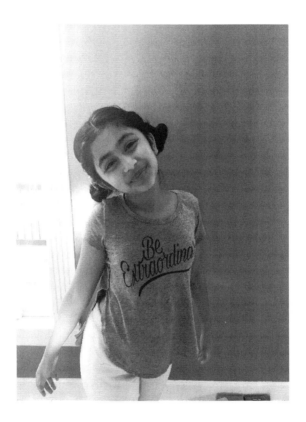

CHAPTER 4:
IMPACTS DURING LOCKDOWN

T he whole world is experiencing the HUGE negative impacts of COVID-19. People's health is at high risk, so there are restrictions in our lives to ensure safety and protection. Hundreds and thousands of people are dying every day. Covid-19 testing facilities are increasing day by day. People are doing self-quarantine to minimize the spread. Governments are working hard to help people in need, providing additional healthcare services, and other financial help. I am going to focus on the following impacts on me as a kid and probably most of the world as the pandemic went on.

1. **Online School:** I knew that I didn't have school because of the virus so does that mean I don't have work? After the weekend ended, it was that Sunday night that I discovered that I had online school and that I had to attend a Zoom meeting

bright and early on Monday. I had no idea what to expect.

a. I woke up at 8:30 to get ready for the Zoom meeting at 9:00 am. Turns out that the Zoom call was pretty good and we talked about the virus, wanting to go back to school.

b. Here is our kickoff conversation. I don't have the exact dialogue so I will just tell you the process of the conversation. My teacher started off the meeting by talking about having no school and then we went onto the topic of homework and normal schoolwork and that's when we got to the part when we discussed online school. Our teacher talked us through on how we would get into Google Classroom and how we would see all the different classroom files and etc. So, we got on and knew what we needed to accomplish and that's how online school went. During NTI (Non-Traditional Instruction), we used to get homework to finish that we would then upload for our teacher to review. I struggled to finish my work in the beginning, especially because I was not focused. Eventually I got better in making and following schedules.

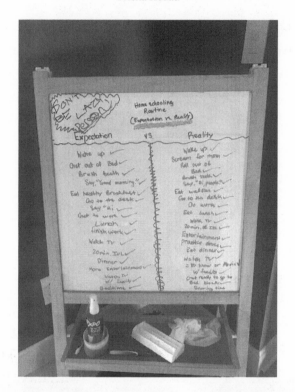

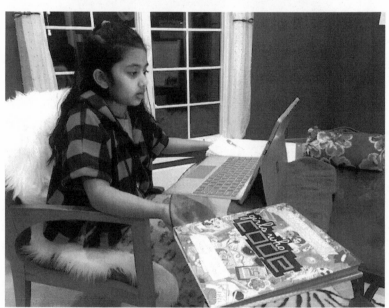

2. **Online Shopping:** As we were social distancing, we obviously couldn't go to the mall. How were we going to shop? We ended up buying things from Amazon, Instacart, and other online venues. It was confusing at the beginning to shop online for food, but it got easier as we did it more often and we are still doing it. I miss going out for shopping with my family, the little treats, and simply being able to go out, and have a normal life. I pointed out that I would be turning ten and my parents gave me some money to spend on Amazon as we wouldn't be going to the store to get what we would want to get. My parents give me some dollars if I finish certain task as a reward and they let me use it my way (with their permission of course). This time, they said I could buy whatever I wanted, within a limit. If I tell you the limit, you are going to freak out! So, sadly, I will not be telling you the limit, but I am excited and have my list ready.

3. **Silent City -** Schools, buildings, and basically the entire city were all closed. One thing I can tell you for sure is that this stuff gets you freaked out. Buildings and schools were closed including mine, and where my parents work. As I said, basically everything you needed was either on

the computer or in your house. Now, who knows when schools will re-open? When will my school re-open? When can we have or normal lives back?

4. **Lockdown** - Another important thing to mention is the DREADFUL lockdown! So, you probably noticed that I live in Kentucky and the city I live in and slowly the state and the whole country went into lockdown. I am not complaining, because this became very serious. I may be nine, but I am much more than that. I know for a fact that this was a pandemic and that it came from a village that apparently is unfortunate. Imagine all those people who are now homeless, lost jobs, are sick, or need help, love, care, and courage. My meaning is to understand how they are feeling it, and the difficulties standing by it. Right now, I am behind the computer trying to find the right word. Champion? Awesome? Cool? Unbeatable? Outstanding? Well, as I said, most of the world on Earth is in lockdown or quarantine. It is important to pay attention to the news because that's the best you could get out of it. I know for a fact that most of the world will not be roaming like a bird to investigate in each and every country. The easier way is watching the new, which I know can be overwhelming. Even kids should know

the latest health and safety information. How many people have the virus? What safety precautions are needed to be followed? How many people are going to be tested? What's the impact on the world other than me? All the answers are either on the news or internet. By the way, did you notice that the Spanish Flu started in the ending of 1917 and beginning of 1918.Which is around 1920 and a hundred years later in 2020 another pandemic started?

5. **Social Distancing:** A big part of ending a pandemic is social distancing and wearing masks. The reason to do this is that if we don't, then there is a very high chance that more people will get infected and more people will die. That's basically why we are doing lockdown and I have to admit that it is boring and sometimes super frustrating but when everybody does their part, the pandemic will start to fade and everyone can get back to normal life. If most people do not do their part, then it's going to take longer and longer. So please wear those masks if you are going outside and do your part. If you are doing your part, then remember that you rock and also remember to hold on tight.

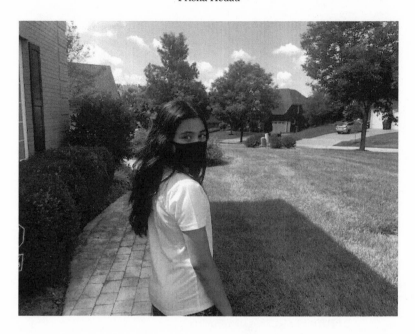

6. **No In-Person Gatherings:** Since social distancing must continue, we can't have large gatherings with friends and family. I think we can now have small gatherings from five to ten people, but still, really not gathering people. On my bed, I have pillows like every other person, but one of the pillows says GATHER. There is a reasoning behind that but that's not my point. You also may have noticed that I enjoy simple and fun gatherings (you know what type of fun that means) so right now this sucks, but it is what it is, I guess.

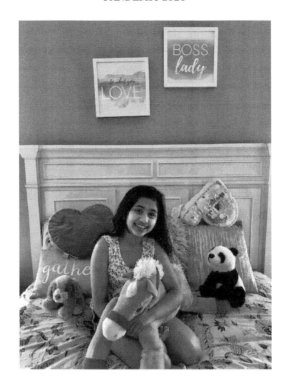

7. **Virtually meet on Google Duo, Zoom, and Google meets:** Last today, but definitely not least, is virtual and online calls. Remember the cousins of my own who live in Europe? Well, right know if there was no pandemic and coronavirus drama, then I would be in Europe, my dream destination, enjoying the view and hanging out with my family. At least we are able to call them and chat for however long we all would like and that's honestly the best part of having a pandemic covering your life like a blanket.

Before social distancing started, I was happy. At this point in the story, however, I wasn't really sure of what I thought about it. We wouldn't be in this self-isolation for that long, right? Wrong. Now new things got my mind flipping because we had to do online grocery shopping? We had to stay six feet apart from everybody, the whole city is closed, etc. Can it really get that bad? I remember at the beginning of the pandemic, we would watch the news and we used to watch Kentucky's governor talking about positive things and giving Kentucky status on the virus, including what precautions to take, information on testing, how many positive cases there were, how it was impacting areas in the world and more.

It got stressful at times and I couldn't have sleepovers, family and friends gatherings, and we couldn't go to the mall. I am pretty healthy and enjoy homemade food, but not going to fast-food restaurants for more than four months is harder than you would think. Also imagine not being able to get to your favorite ice cream shop! Life was getting scary and boring and people were panicking before adjusting to the new normal.

CHAPTER 5:
THINGS TO DO DURING QUARANTINE

Here is an example of a normal day in a pandemic. Good Morning Prisha, it's 9:45 am. Go downstairs to brush your teeth and eat breakfast. All full? Now you can go watch some tv. Do something random for a while or finish work than you can go upstairs. One hour later, I go all the way downstairs to practice for the next dance. Oh, it's been an hour, lunch time! Yum! That is called a good lunch, right there. Now walk on the deck with mom. Then there is time to do whatever, such as watch television, read a book, draw or chalk the sidewalk, call grandparents, etc. Soon, however, I realized with the help of my parents that it is not working. I have built a schedule for myself with the things I like to do for fun, or a hobby along with two hours of study time daily. This really helped me stay on top of things. I also found time to pick up my hobbies. I am sharing details, hoping this will give you some idea to organize your own routine while having fun, and learning new things.

Remember to do social distancing. This is about maintaining safe distance with others while you are around other people (including you) safe. My parents and I are very serious and take all the safety precautions to social distance. We stay ten to twelve feet apart from everybody, we wear our masks, and make sure that we are not touching our faces and washing hands regularly.

Have a schedule of what you like. As I mentioned in my intro, I have my own YouTube channel. I spent time preparing dance or other material to share with everyone. I like dancing a lot, so I practice dance regularly. Dance is something that takes time to master and I can't say that I am a professional, but I do try to make it look like I am. No dancer can be good if she or he doesn't practice. My dad always says focus on quality, not quantity. I agree with him. I practice every day a little by little so I can post those videos. Do whatever you like, but practice discipline and dedication towards that to keeps yourselves busy and be productive.

Calling Friends: I miss meeting my friends a lot during quarantine. We are social distancing so we can't go and meet friends or see them at school. Calling them once in a while is something very nice and I love seeing them. It's not just friends, but family and others as well. Google Duo, Google Meets, and Zoom calls keep you busy and makes you happy when you see the faces of people you love the most. Staying connected is very important during times like this.

Helping out in the household work: While we are stuck at the home, it is nice to help out your parents with little things. Sometimes it's as simple as folding clothes or helping in making a meal with mom or dad. I also enjoy setting dinner tables or little stuff like that.

My mom acts like that house comes with a big price and a big load of work and she is not wrong.

I'd say that if you are not disciplined and always on track like me, then in quarantine you might get more productive or become a lazy brat. Though I am not a brat, I am getting pretty lazy many times, so staying active is a must. To stay active I dance, run around our lake, walk, chalk drawing, and help out. I basically just listed everything that I mentioned before this sentence and right now if you are thinking why I said I am lazy and I still do all of

that work. The answer is that parents shouldn't underes-
timate me. I am not totally lazy.

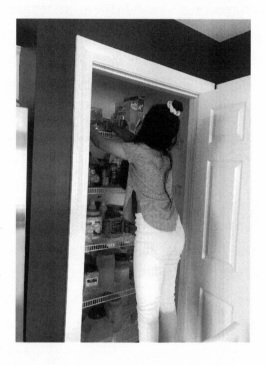

Watching TV News: Watching some TV and
the news, especially the news, is pretty important right now —especially the soccer station.
It is pretty important, because you can keep
track of the world and now what will happen
and what can happen next. What precautions
should we take? When will lockdown end? Is
the vaccine out yet? Most of the answer will be
on the news.

Baking: This is a new hobby I picked up during the pandemic. I've started out by helping and now enjoy doing baking with my mom Me and my mom, or sometimes even my dad, bake—banana bread, cookies, pizza, and more. With my dad, I baked his childhood favorite cake of his mom's recipe and it came out pretty good. I thought the cake was going to burn for sure, but we were lucky, I guess! My point is, exploring new things is important. It also made me realize that I can bake sometimes.

Cooking: Cooking was something we do every day at home. We prefer vegetarian homemade food. We love homemade food but don't mind premade food or frozen food works sometimes. Cooking was not too exciting for me, but it was something that kept me busy for a while. It is not easy or my most favorite things to do, but I could spend time with my parents so I helped anyway. You can try as well!

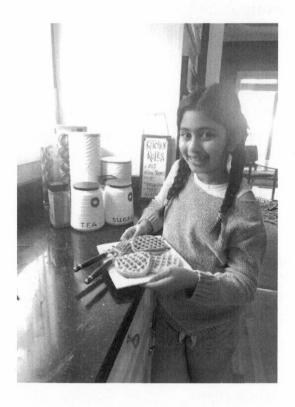

Homemade Smoothies: I LOVE smoothies in summer. We try making a lot of smoothies using fresh and frozen fruits. One was a berry smoothie with blueberries, raspberries, strawberries, and blackberries. That's a lot of berries! Another one was a cherry and mango smoothie with a scoop of vanilla ice-cream on top. Yum! My dad and I tried it, but my mom was not a big fan and complained about how much sugar it contained.

Painting:

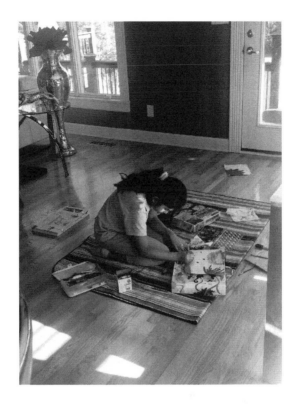

CHAPTER 6:
TIPS FOR ONLINE SCHOOLING

I'd share a few tips if it would be helpful for the people that will be doing online school. Let's go one by one:

Study Desk: First off—you should have a comfortable seating area for you while you study because you will be there most of the day. It is extremely important to have a designated area in your house. If you keep moving from place to place, it will disturb the people around you and sooner or later will distract you, so it's always good to find one area.

> **Be presentable:** If you have online school, Zoom call, or any other meeting classes, you are always expected to be presentable. This means your clothes should be decent, but also, make sure their comfortable and you can wear them all day long. Second, the scenery behind you should be decent not catchy.

Consider having a plain or simple wall behind you. Having few frames, or a little decoration won't hurt. Make sure that you are not in a spot where you know for a fact that that it will not work. Customize it the way you like it to have easy access to the supplies and avoid distractions. I like to keep books on one side and a pencil pouch and other things on the other.

Discipline: This is something very important, and if you don't have discipline you will struggle (for sure). I don't have much discipline but I am working on it. The next points will help you with it in case you are like me.

A Schedule: As I said, if you aren't much into discipline, then you need your parents help to make a schedule for yourself. Once you have that, try to stick with that. In my case, if I follow the schedule or complete a task, I get rewards from my parents—little things like ice cream, money for piggy bank etc. That works for me to stay motivated. This is like your sidekick, so try it out but let me tell you that it may take some time to get used to and you will also need encouragement to follow the schedule.

Finishing your work on time: Sometimes finishing work can be overwhelming especially when you get behind. It is always a good idea to finish a task on time and having a daily routine. Don't forget to submit back online so your teacher can review. Your schedule can help in this job even if you are discipline. If you have a planner, please go ahead and use that.

Collaboration: This brings us to self-patience. When you are on a group call, or in your online classes it is important to collaborate with everyone. This will help your friends/not-so-friends /classmates because they might be struggling and want to ask a question or help. Working together is FUN, but you need to be intentional and work as a TEAM. You will be happy and relieved after the job and the extra work is done!

Raise your hand: Give the people in your calls or a class a sign before you start talking to make sure you are not cutting off someone. This will also allow teachers and students to work better together. Don't be shy, speak up, and ask questions and offer help.

Be Mindful: Being mindful is always good. We all are different and sometimes not aware about other's situation so starting by asking how people are doing is a good thing.

CHAPTER 7:
FOCUS ON THE POSITIVE THINGS

As you know, I complained about a few different things in my book, spoke about my struggles, but also shared the tips that helped me embrace the new normal of this life. While this is not an ideal situation for any one of us, I am taking an opportunity to share the little I have accomplished this year during the pandemic to focus on the positivity. I am so hopeful that it will end soon. Cross your fingers, not four just two of them!

This year has been great and has given me a lot of new life experiences. Thank you, 2020, but also, No Thanks. I tried my best to stay happy, busy, and not get lost during these certain times. My parents always root for me and give me the values and love that each kid deserves.

Something I would like to add right here is that I am not trying to show off or brag in any way. Keeping a list of your own achievements and looking back is always helpful. I started doing this recently, and refer back for self-talking, my readers. I suggest you do the same to make the most of your time and feel good about it.

This year started off with celebrating mor than one hundred subscribers on my YouTube channel (Channel name: Prisha Hedau). This was a pretty nice accomplishment for me. I do videos for fun, but some people took the time to subscribe and support me and for that I am very thankful. I have recorded a couple of videos to support the COVID situation, involving cooking and dancing. Go Subscribe and explore more about me!

I play chess at state level. Do you know only a few girls play Chess? We had tournaments until January. I won a couple of games and title trophies for chess. I have been doing chess and going to tournaments for about three and a half years now and participated in the All Girls USA National Chess Championships in Chicago. I slowly made my way up to the USA National top 100 players for Girls age 7 and under. (I secured sixtieth position overall in March 2018).

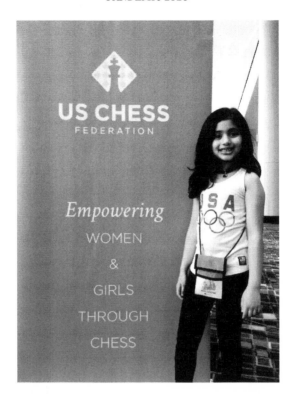

I was in fourth grade this year and ended it success-fully with all A's and I was pretty happy because fourth grade was a big change after third grade. This year I tried Math Kangaroo and got a whopping result of sev-enth rank in the state of Kentucky and twenty-first in the U.S.A. National ranking. These small things I man-aged to learn and earn this year. That makes me happy because I worked hard for it.

I'm almost becoming two digits in age! (Yay, ten in September). I have become a good video editor and so I do my own editing for my YouTube channel. I am on my school STLP (Student Technology Leadership Program), which helped me learn new computer skills. I do swimming for fun and as an exercise. I missed it a lot this year. We don't have a swimming pool at our home and classes are closed due to COVID-19. I made my way up to a level higher this year working with my coach. Water makes me happy, pool water and sides of beaches not in the middle of the ocean.

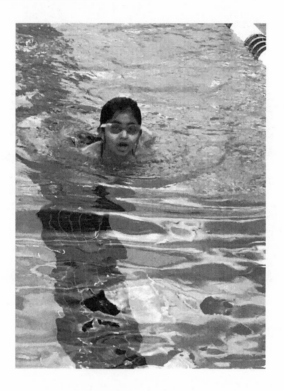

CHAPTER 8:
LESSONS LEARNT

Health is Wealth: During this health crisis, it is extremely important to take care of your health and I don't mean working out five hours straight or doing intense yoga. I am trying to say that small things you do to take care of your health will make a big difference. You might even start the good habit and help yourself a ton in the future. If you are healthy, you can beat anything in life. I would like to add that if you need to go to the doctor during the pandemic, you should not have an excuse. You should take a lot of precautions, but this is something you really don't want to avoid.

I walk a lot and sometimes even run, which helps me and my body. I feel good after exercising, and I feel relieved. Sometimes I do yoga with my mom. Dancing is my hobby, and if you don't want to work out or do yoga, dancing for one to two hours will still help you. Do sleep well.

Eating Healthy: I eat two to three serving of fruits and veggies in a day, and also plenty of milk, I try to eat mostly healthfully. My cheat list includes cookies, ice-cream, and donuts. I am not a super healthy eater, but I try my best. My parents do a good job reminding me of the importance of nutrition in food. Well do you know how to read a food label? If not, ask your parents. There is a lot of sugar, sodium, etc. in many pre-packaged foods.

Be Happy: The last piece of advice I have to offer is that you should always find ways to keep your brain active, busy, and fresh. For example, if things are stressing you out, which is easy to happen during a pandemic, calling your friends will keep you happy and will refresh your brain.

Safety guidelines: Follow safety guidelines to protect yourself and others. Wearing a mask and social distancing helps greatly with limiting the virus spread. Avoid crowed places, vacations, large gathering etc. Stay healthy at home!

Technology is a saver: I am sure you all agree to this. We can't imagine our lives without internet, phone, or video calls. I knew technology is everywhere in our life but my appreciation for technology has reached to another level during this pandemic. Actually, I struggled and learned a few new things this year, for example e.g. Goggle Duo, Zoom, iMovie, Google Docs, Microsoft word, and Power Point. I did take an online class to learn coding and built a simple software mobile application.

Don't Panic: In the beginning of the pandemic, many people got panicked and overstocked a lot of groceries and essential items for their family. A lot of us faced the shortage of the grocery supplies and essential items like toilet paper, hand sanitizers, etc. I remember, we going to different shops and not able to find a toilet paper. The challenge is, many senior people and others in need were struggling to get daily supplies. The lesson I have learned is not to get panicked and then overstock, but be mindful for those around us and need help.

Care about Others: Thinking beyond us is the most important lesson. We as a family do our part to help those in need whether it is a small gesture or a providing support to those in need. I feel happy seeing how many people around the world are helping others. Don't be selfish, take care of yourself, but take care of others too.

Hopefully this gives you some tips for self-care and what can you do to take care for others.

CHAPTER 9:
LOOKING AHEAD

Good job! You are almost done with the book. This is the second to last chapter. In this chapter I will discuss the future, so I hope you Enjoy. Let's Read!

Summer is coming to an end and school is on its way back. My school has made the decision to start school on August 25, 2020 and do Non-Traditional Instructions (NTI) online schooling for the first six weeks. This might change but for now this is what they have announced. It is something I thought was really convenient and nice. My school decided to help arrange the school supplies online so we wouldn't have to struggle and take the risk to go to the stores.

Hopefully COVID-19 will move out of our way in near future, and we will come back to the normal life. I am also very optimistic that someone in this world will find the solution and we will have a vaccine but I don't know. That day would be awesome for all of us. My parents and I discuss our new normal life a lot and how it will be different. Hopefully it will be something that we will all eventually get comfortable living with. I can't wait to meet my friends and classmates again in person and do outdoor activities without taking any precautions.

One of my biggest bucket list items is to run without a mask in the playground with all my friends and hug them without masks, fear, or permission. I didn't know it could be a wish list item but let's face it, it is today's reality.

One other important thing is to help those in need. You can search in google or ask a friend about organizations supporting others. Every little help counts. Me and my family supports DareToCare to do our little part in helping people get meals.

CHAPTER 10:
BE GRATEFUL

Something I would like to add before concluding this book is to live a life of gratitude. I am so grateful that my family and friends are safe because many families have lost someone they love the most. My thoughts are with everyone who faced any loss during this time. I have also learned the importance of small things in life. We do daily prayers because we think that faith and belief goes a long way.

I also want to confess that this job of being an author looked easy at first. Now that I have the experience, I know this job comes with a lot of honesty, determination, and hard work. Now every book that I read and every author I see will be appreciated by me! Thank you for taking your time to read this book. Wish me and the whole world luck. Let the future come our way!

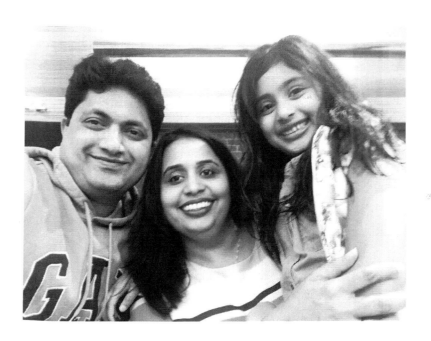